Cardio

Educise
4 Kids
EDUCATION & EXERCISE FOR KIDS

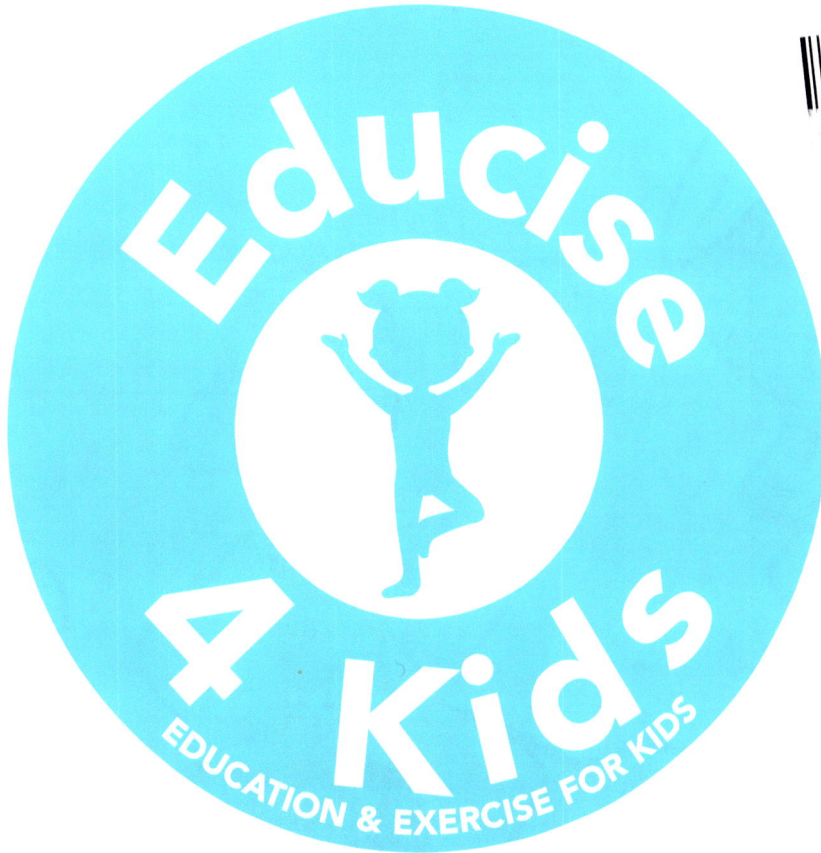

Created By
Priscilla Fauvette

Illustrated By
Bernard Fauvette

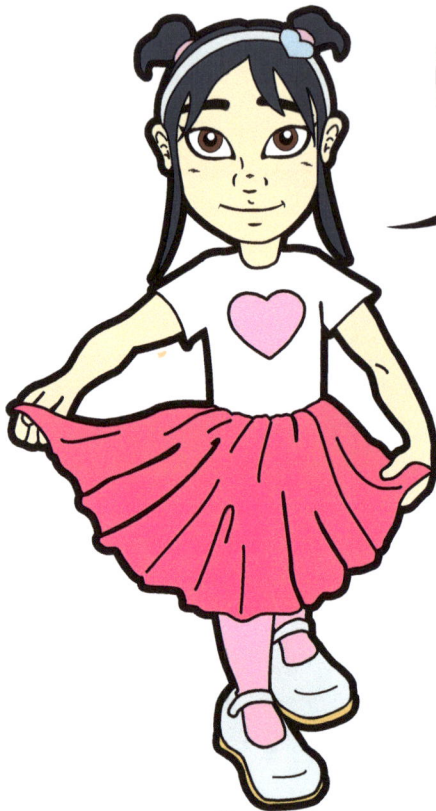

MAKE TIME FOR REST & RELAXATION

LIN

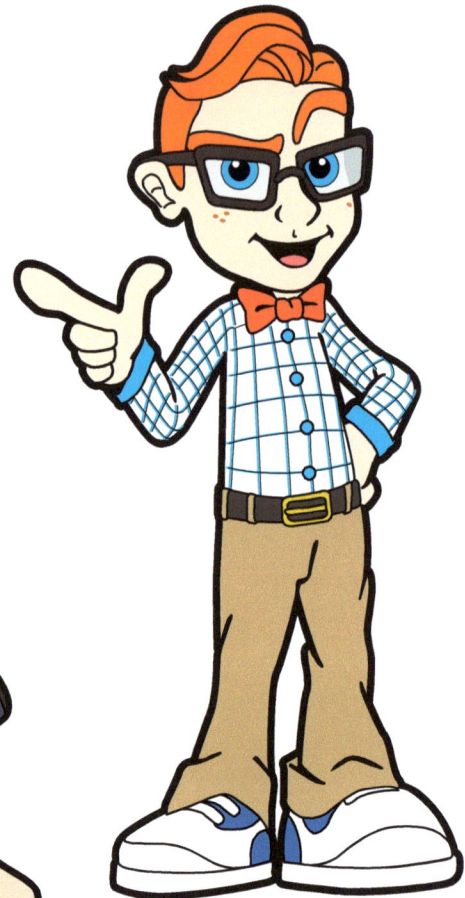

CADEN

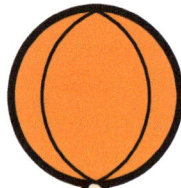

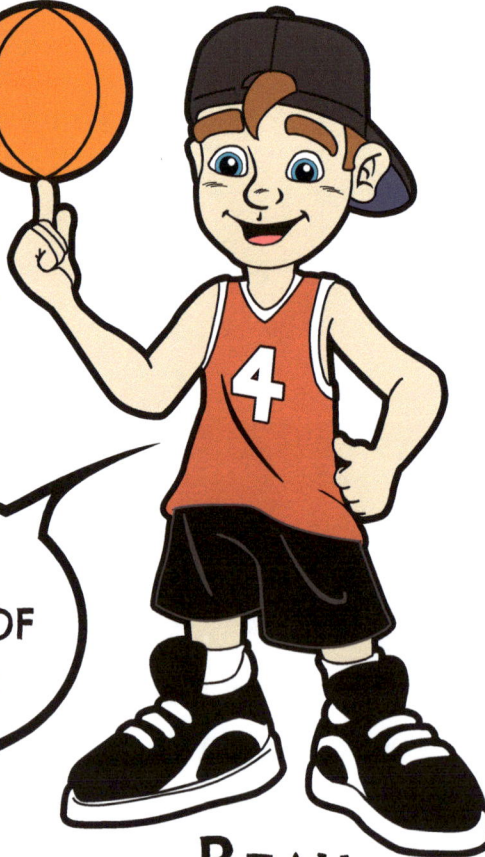

DRINK PLENTY OF WATER

BEAU

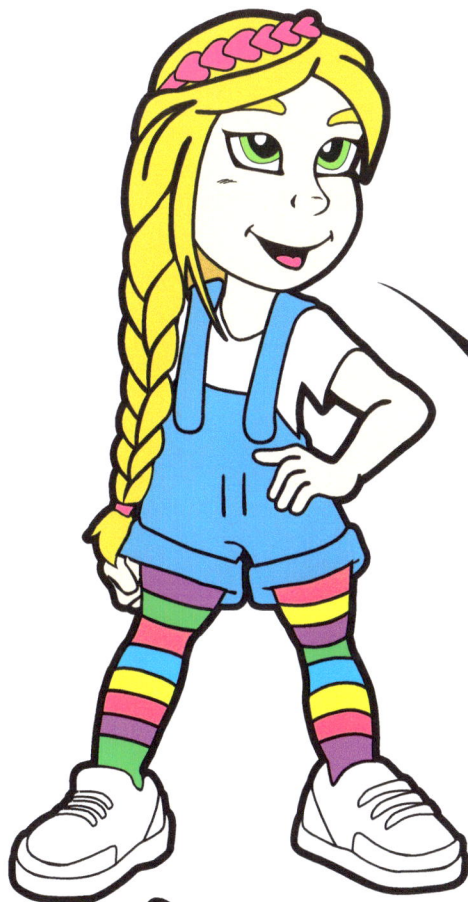

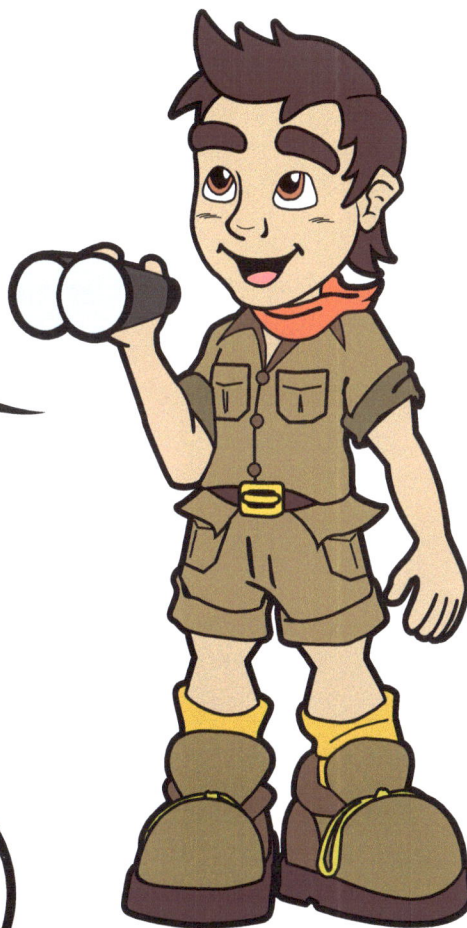

EAT PLENTY OF HEALTHY FOOD

LIMIT SCREEN TIME

MOVE YOUR BODY OFTEN

SOPHIE

ZAC

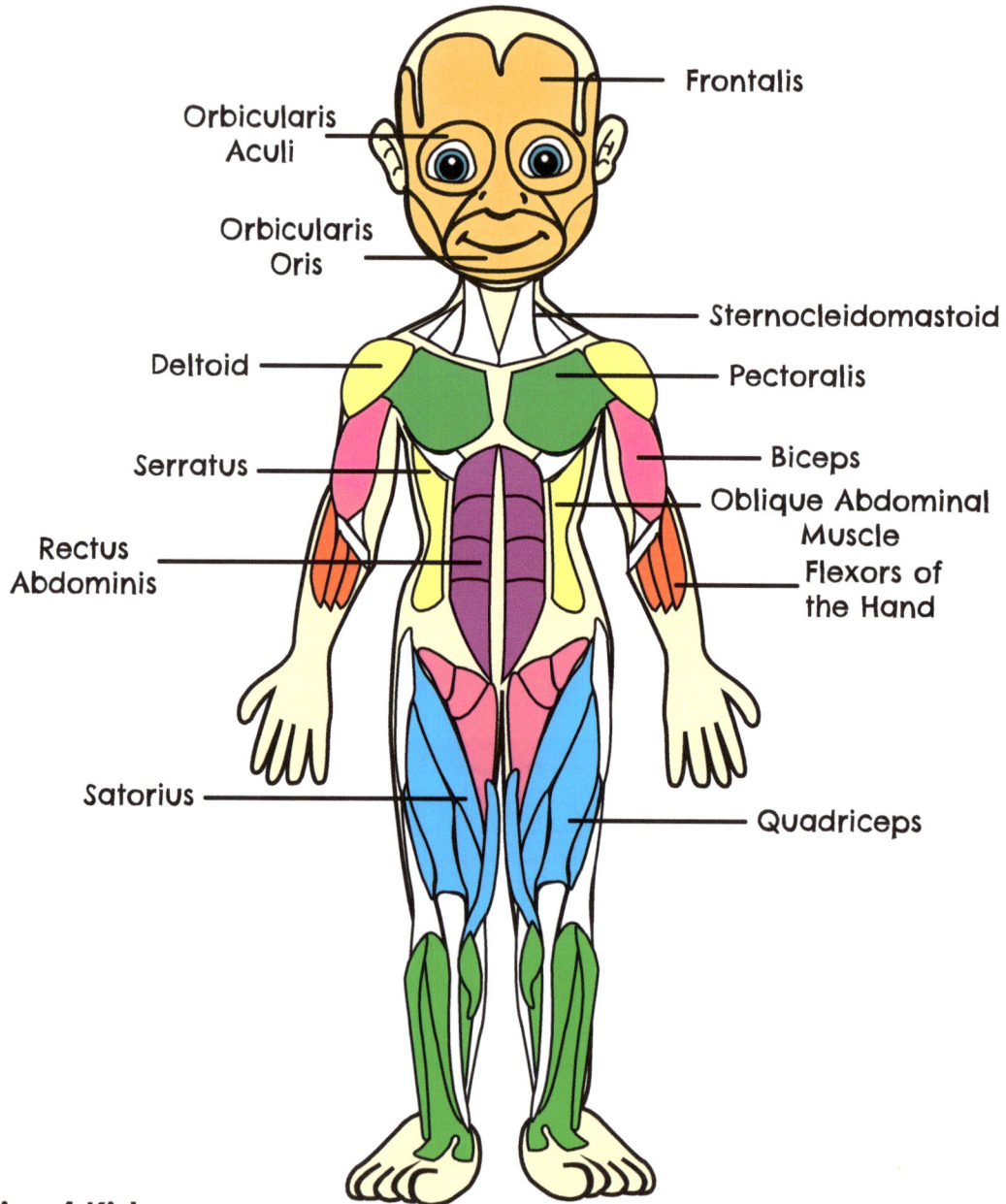

Anatomy

Frontalis

Orbicularis Aculi

Orbicularis Oris

Sternocleidomastoid

Deltoid

Pectoralis

Serratus

Biceps

Oblique Abdominal Muscle

Rectus Abdominis

Flexors of the Hand

Satorius

Quadriceps

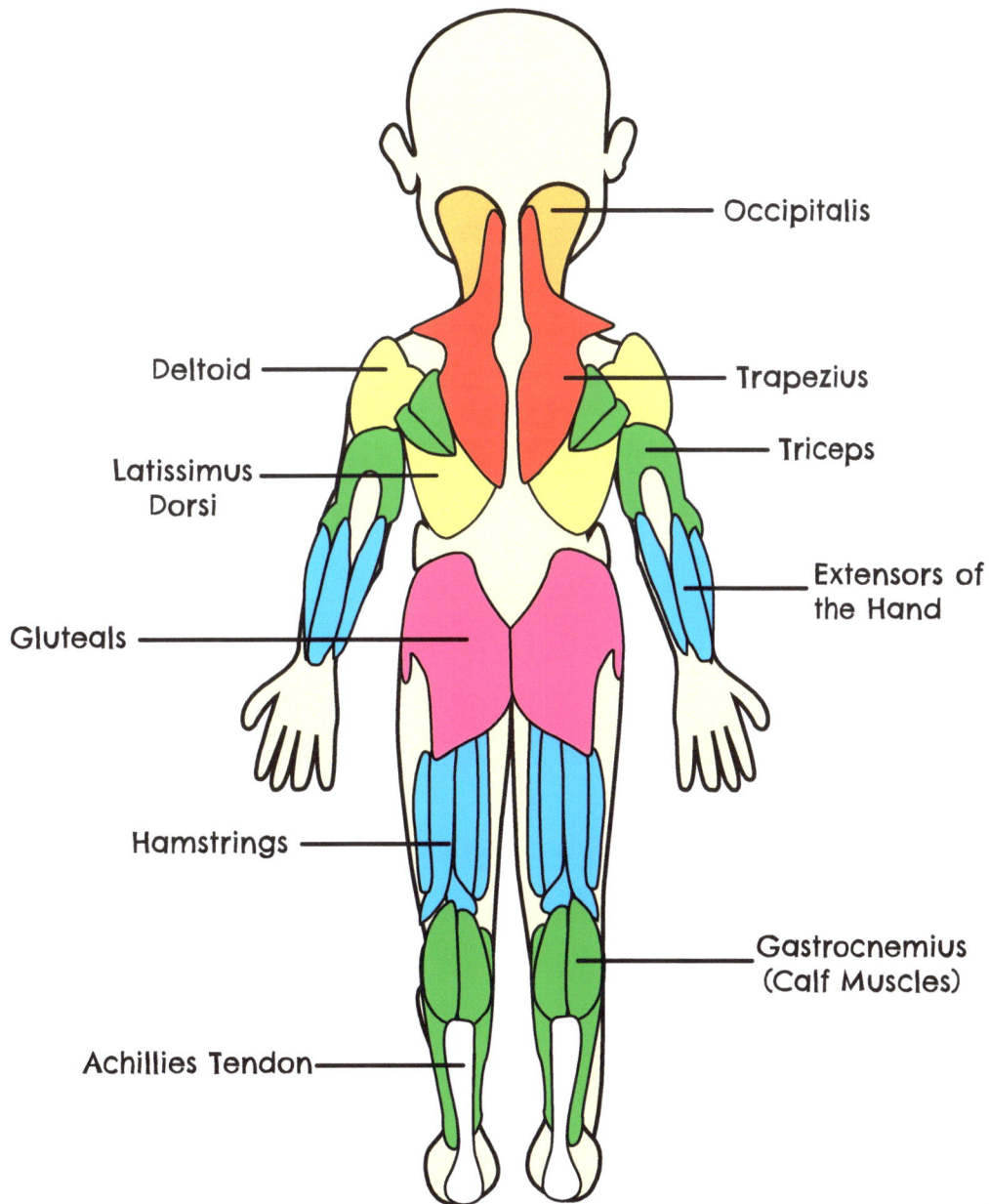

Anatomy

Occipitalis

Deltoid

Trapezius

Triceps

Latissimus
Dorsi

Gluteals

Extensors of
the Hand

Hamstrings

Gastrocnemius
(Calf Muscles)

Achillies Tendon

Straight / Right Punches

Put your gloves on your hands

Stand slightly side on with your body

Bring both hands up near your chin

Punch one arm forward at a time

Can you do this 5 times each side?

1.

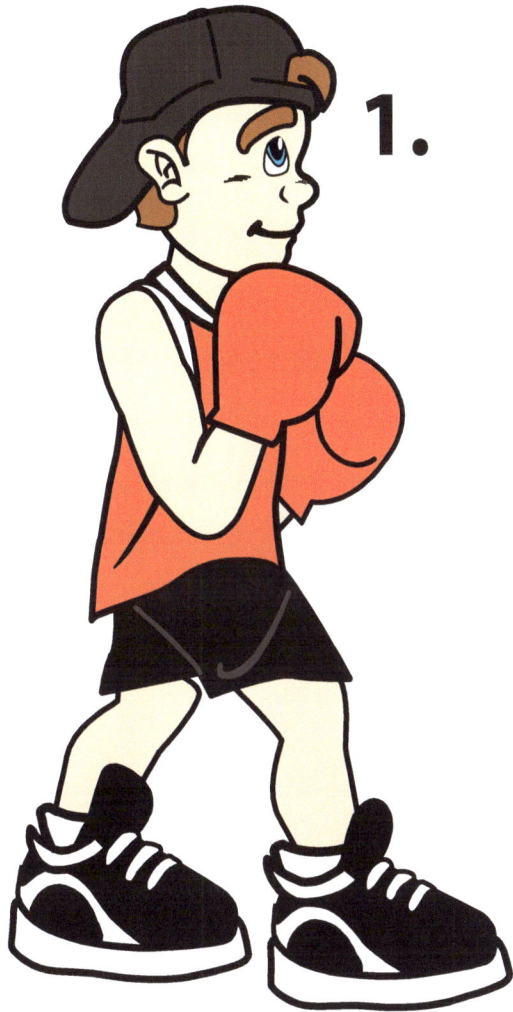

2.

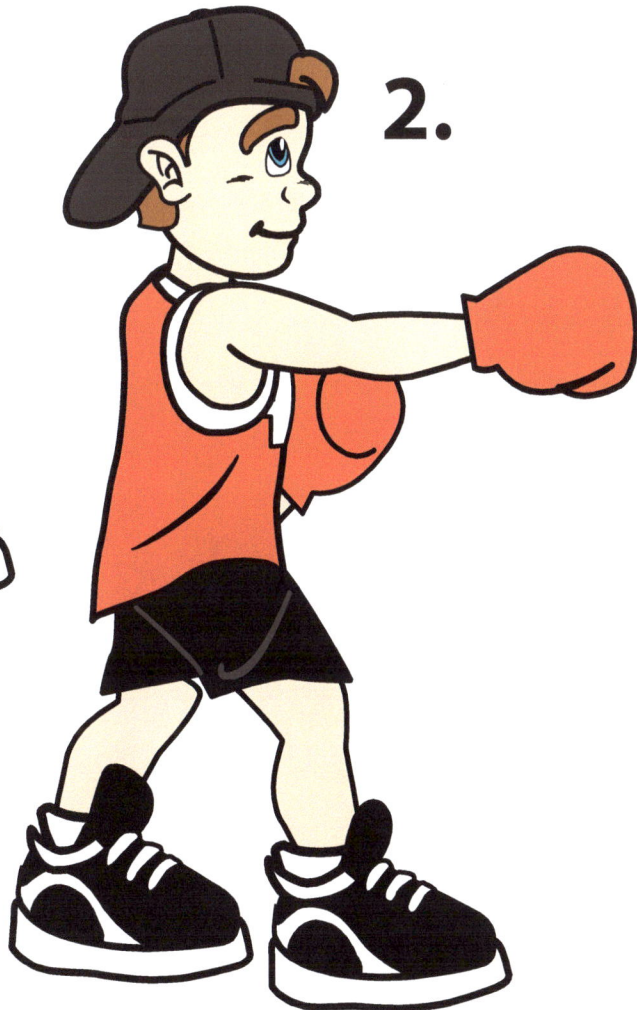

Uppercut Punches

Put your gloves on your hands

Stand slightly side on with your body

Bring both hands up near your chin

Punch one arm upward at a time

Can you do this 5 times each side?

1.

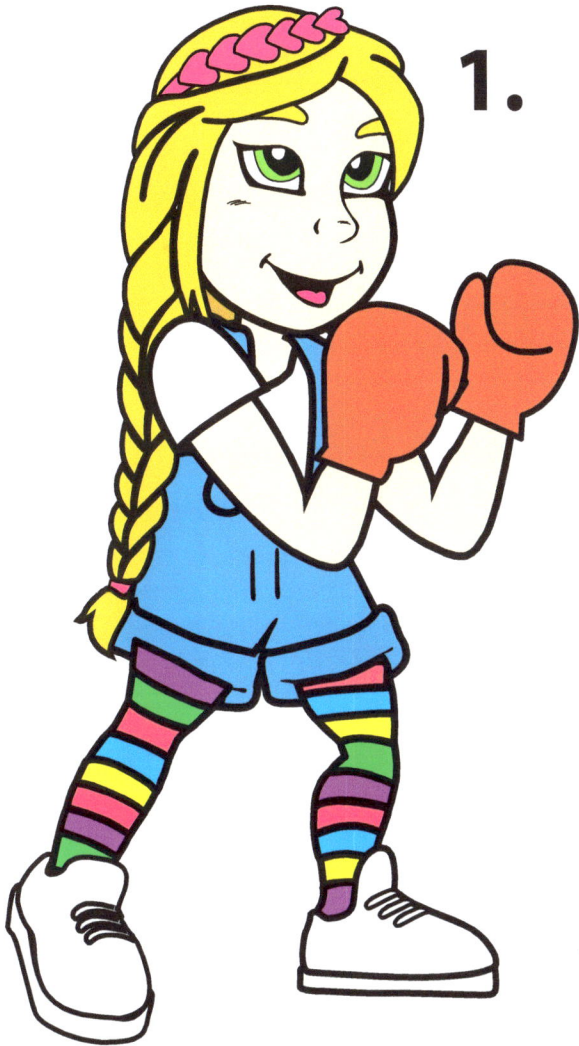

2.

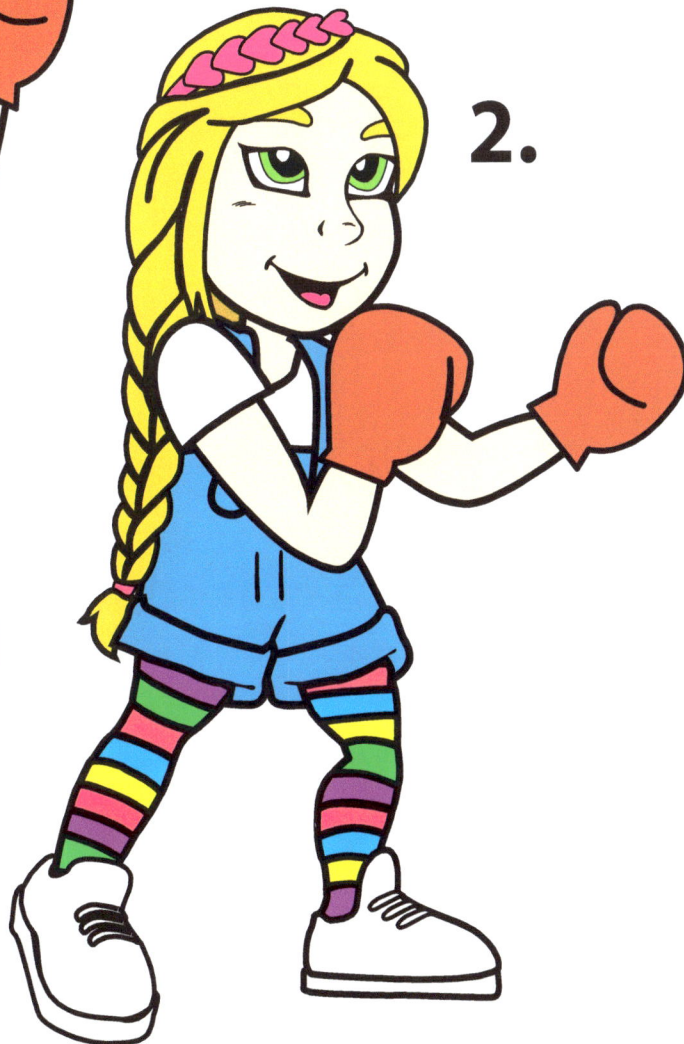

Hopping

Stand up straight and try to
balance on one leg
Bend your arms and start to swing them
forward and backwards
When your arms are back bend your
straight leg a little at the knee
Swing your arms forward and take a
hop at the same time
Can you hop 5 times on each leg?

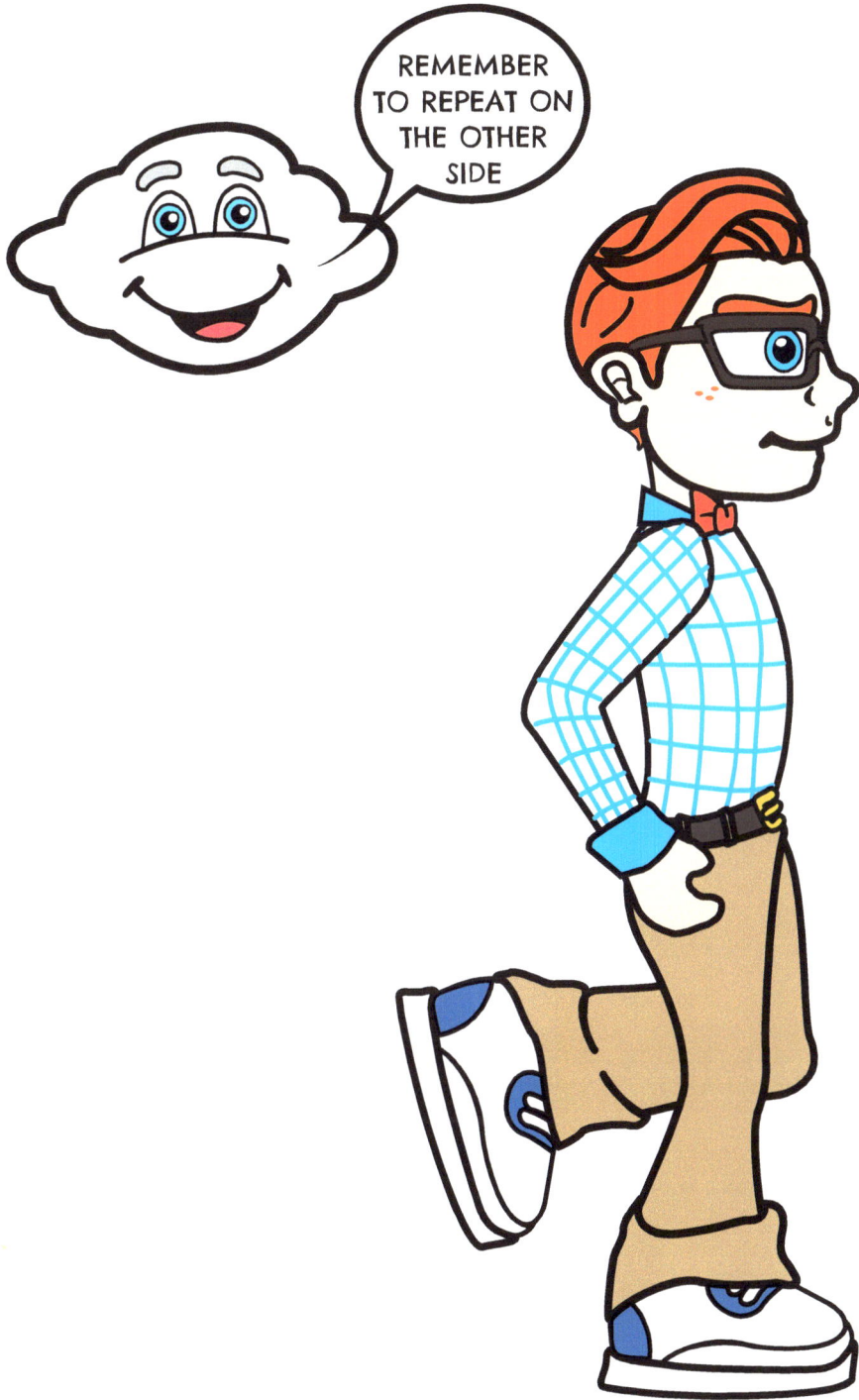

Ski Jumps

Stand up straight
Put your feet apart
Bend your knees slightly
Keep your elbows bent
Swing your arms as you leap from one
foot to the other side to side
Can you do this 5 times each leg?

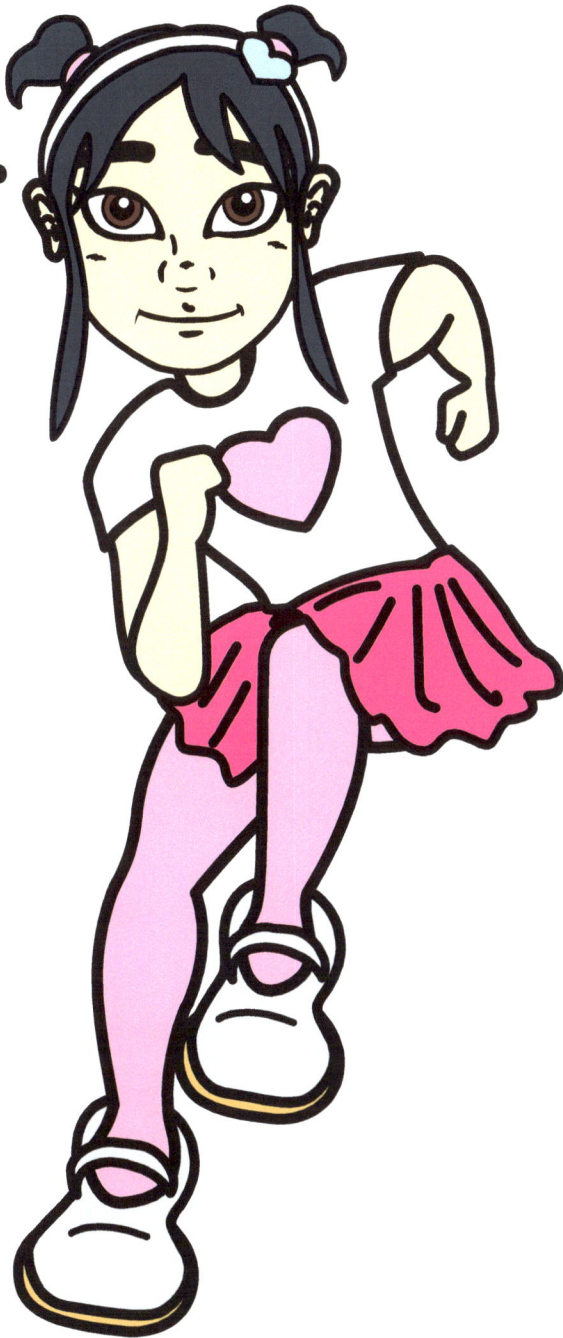

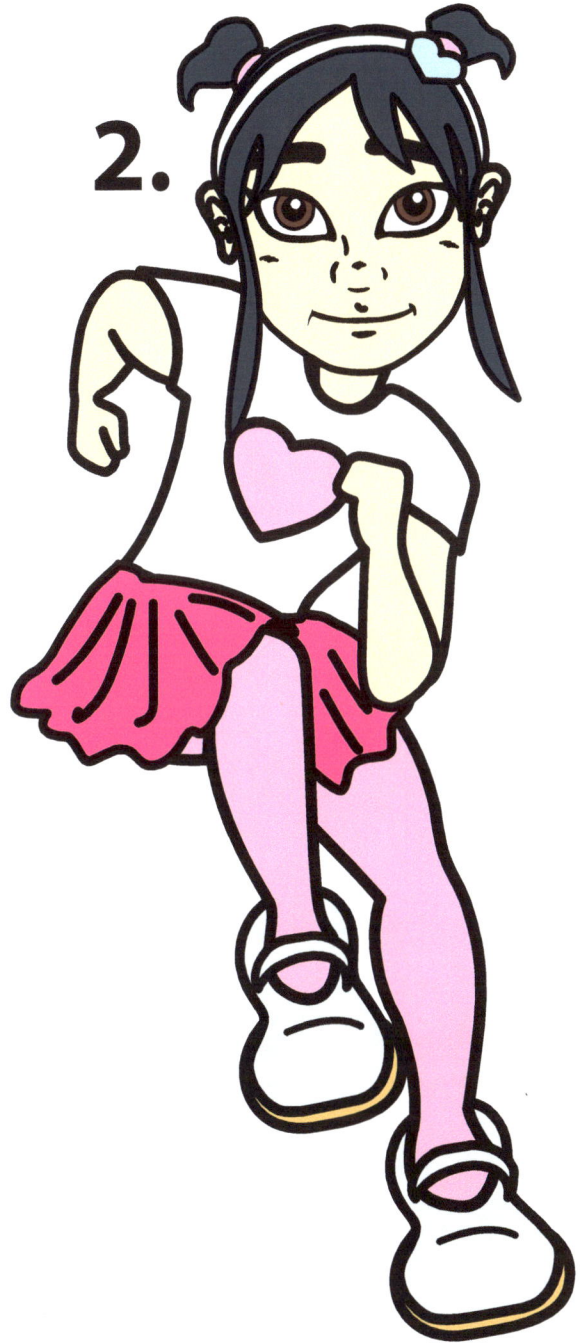

1.

2.

Jump Squats

Stand up straight

Put your feet apart

Bend your knees

Bring your hands back

Spring off your feet

Bring your hands up

Jump as high as you can

Can you do this 5 times?

1.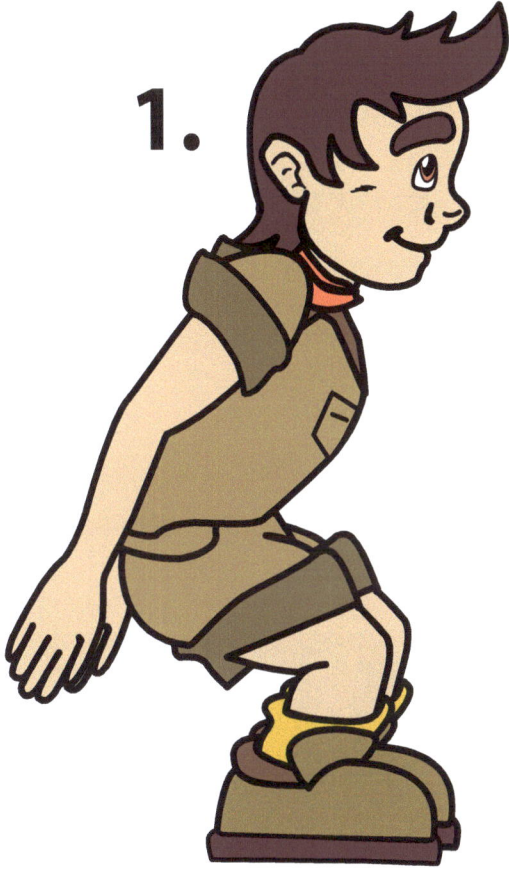

2.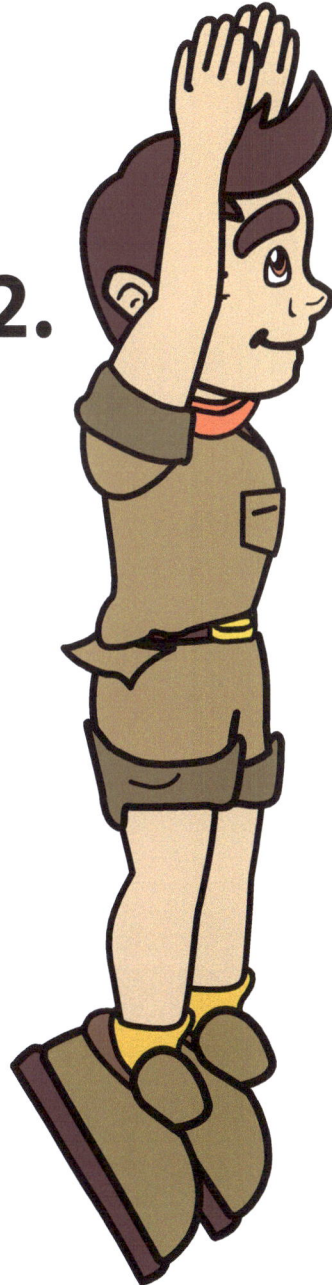

Burpees

Squat down on the floor

Place your hands on the floor

Push your legs straight back

Pull your legs back in

Now jump straight back up with power

Can you do this 5 times?

1.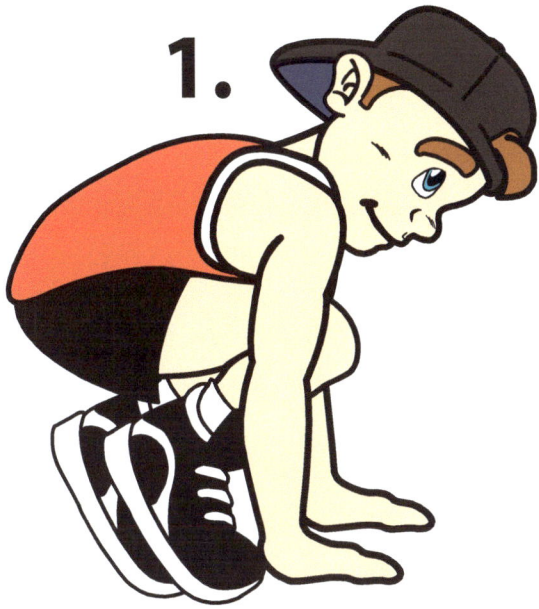

2.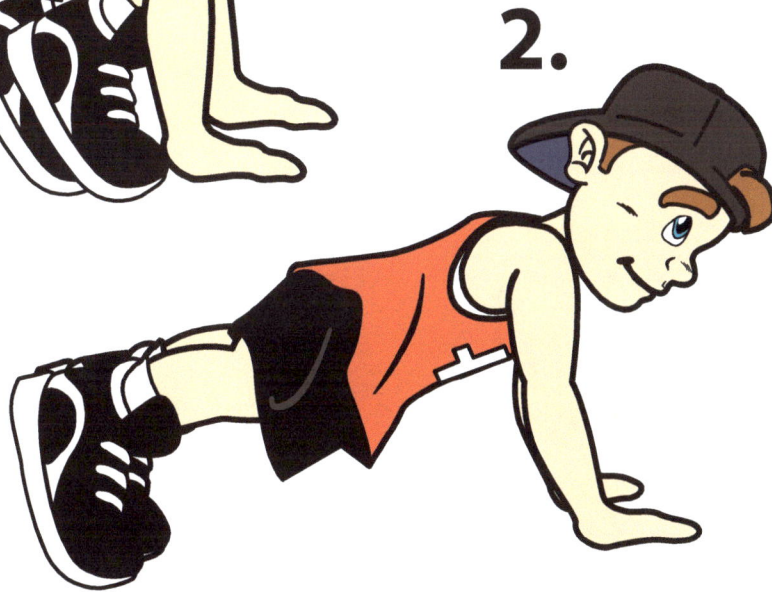

3.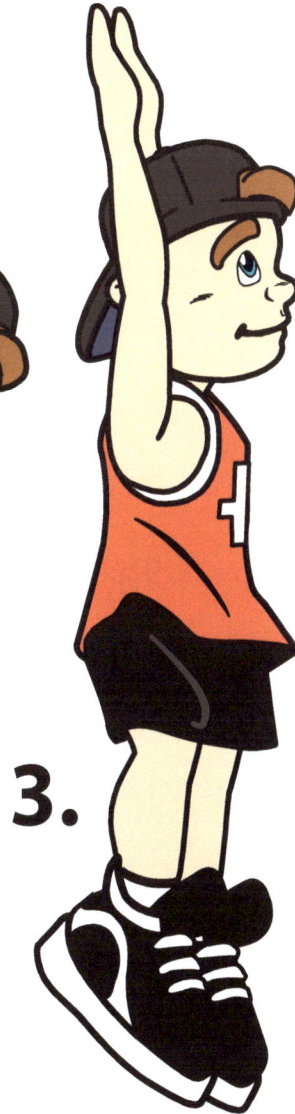

High Knees

Stand with your body straight

Bend your elbows

Start swinging them by your sides hip to lip

Start to lift your knees and jog on the spot

Can you do this 5 times each leg?

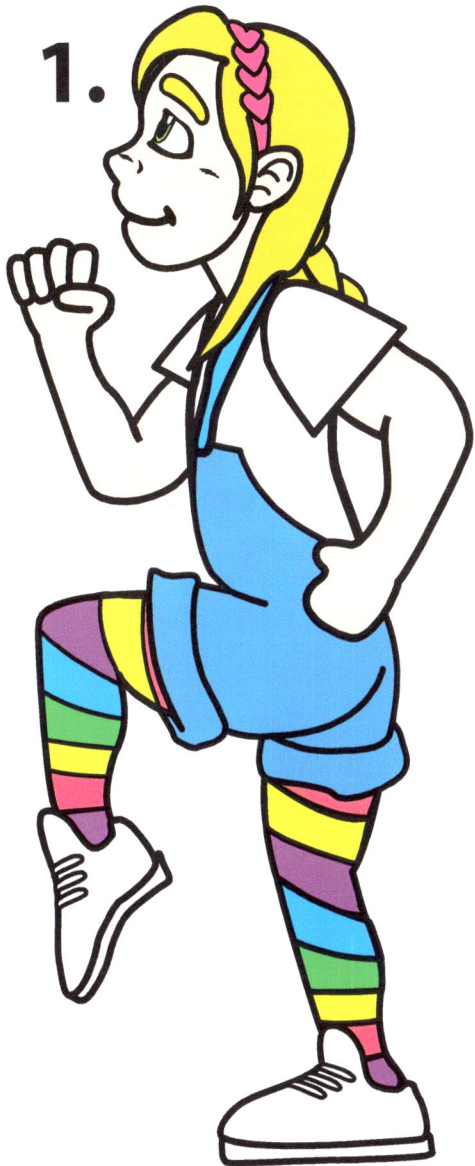

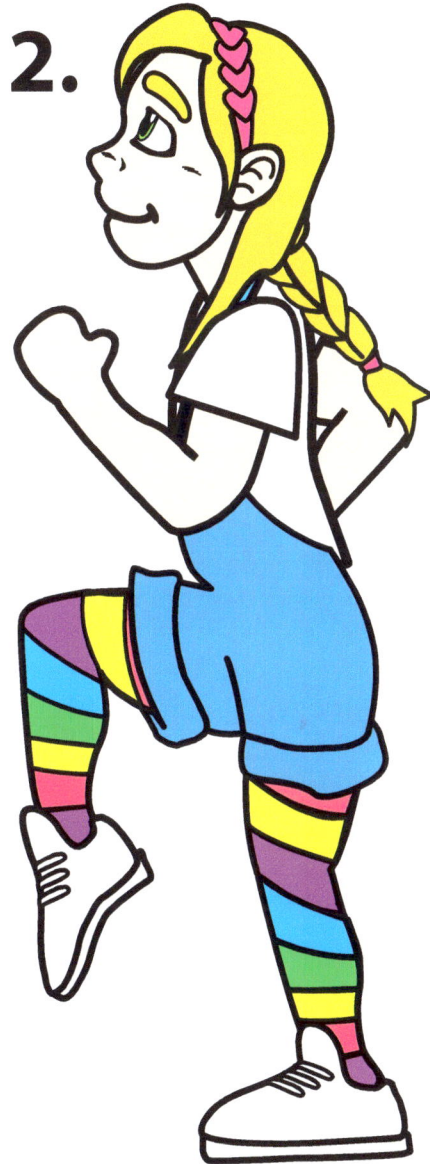

1.

2.

Walking

Let's find a big space

Stand with your body straight

Start slowly swinging your arms by your side

Start to lift your feet

Take small steps forward one leg at a time

Can you walk every day for at least
10 minutes?

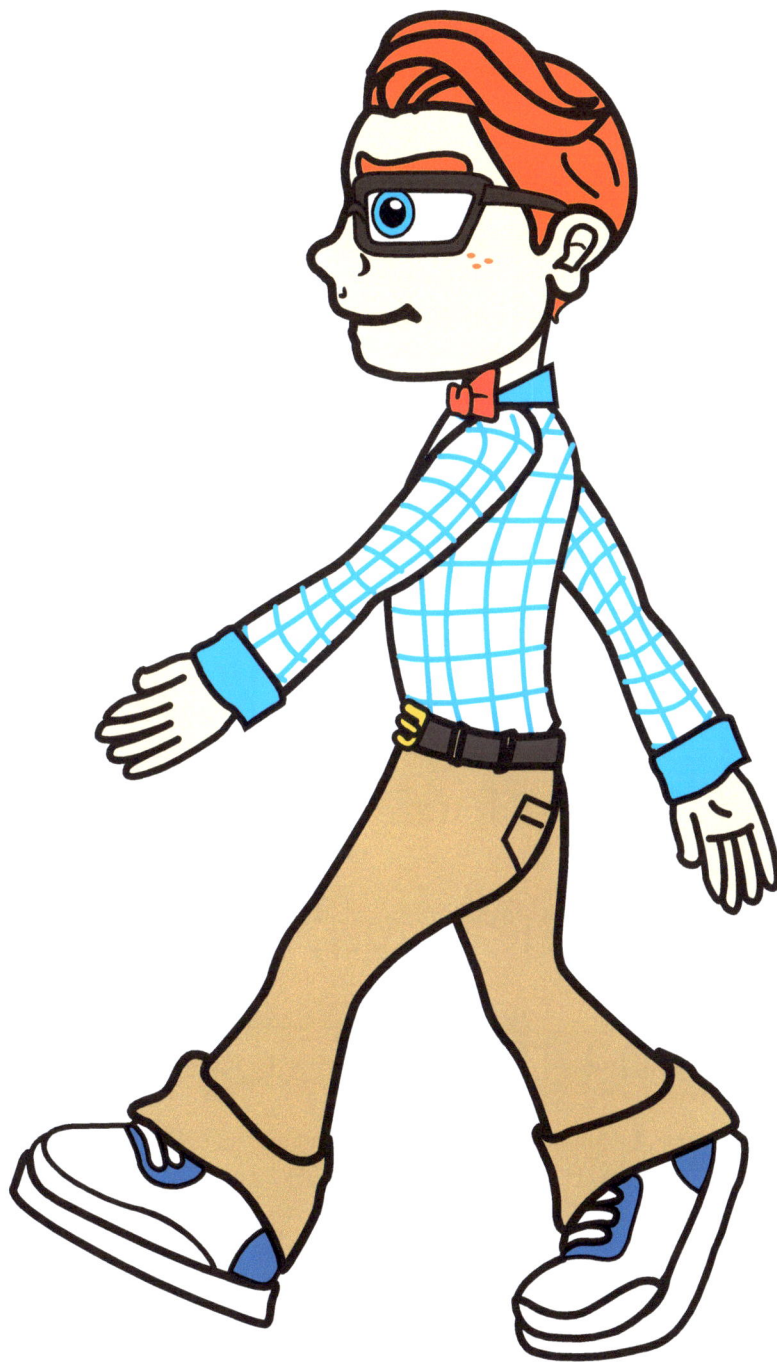

Cardio 21

Star Jumps

Stand up straight

Put your hands by your sides

Take a jump and put your feet and

hands apart at the same time

Bring them out together

Bring them in together

Can you do this 5 times?

1.

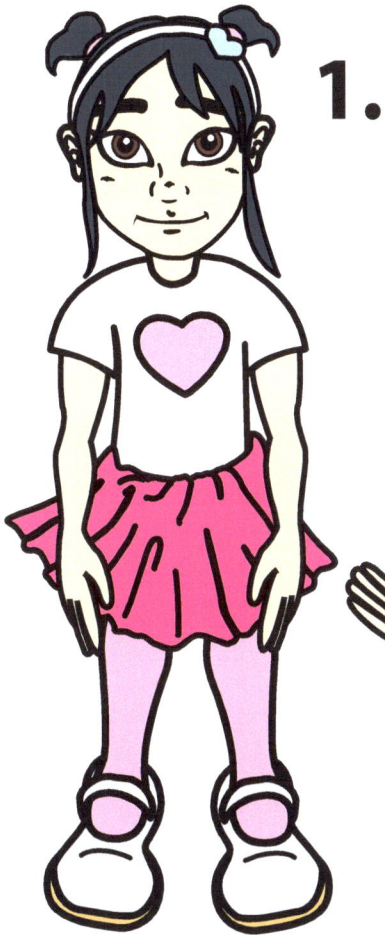

2.

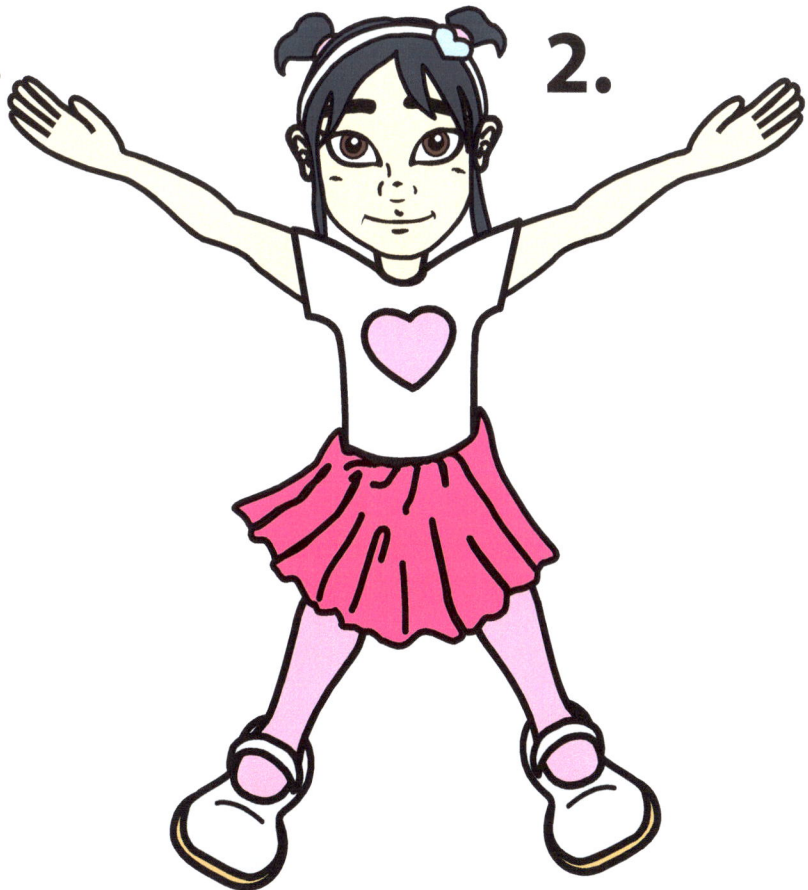

Frog Jumps

Stand up straight

Put your feet apart

Bend your knees

Bring your hands back

Spring off your feet

Bring your hands up

Land softly back on your feet

Can you do this 5 times?

1.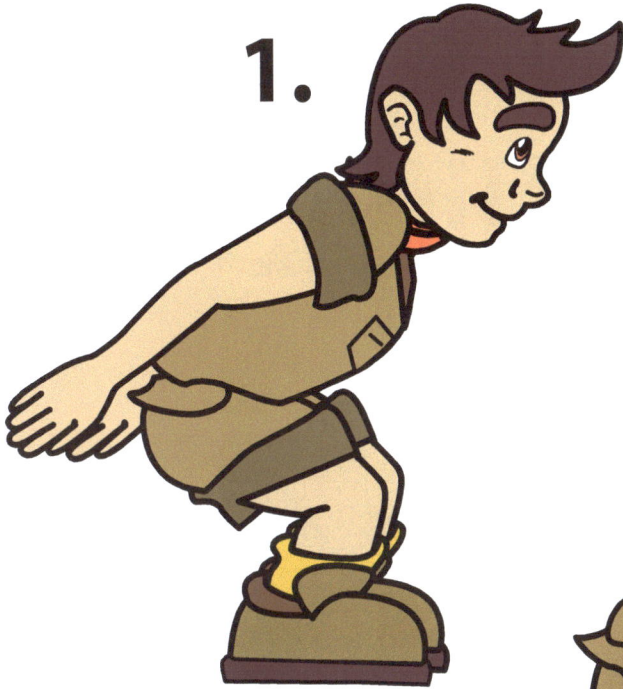

2.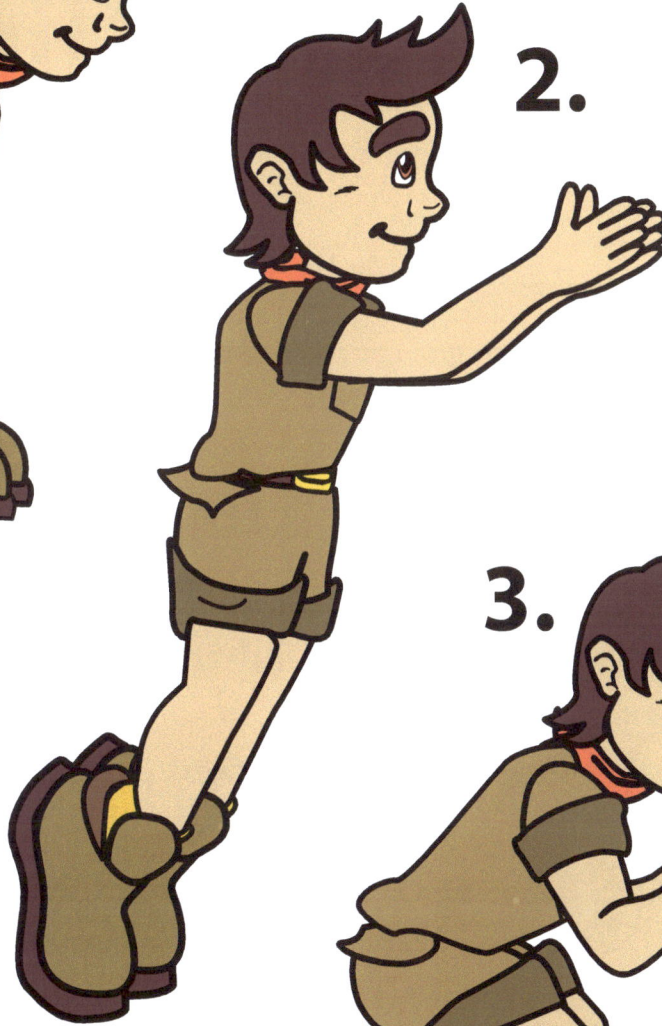

3.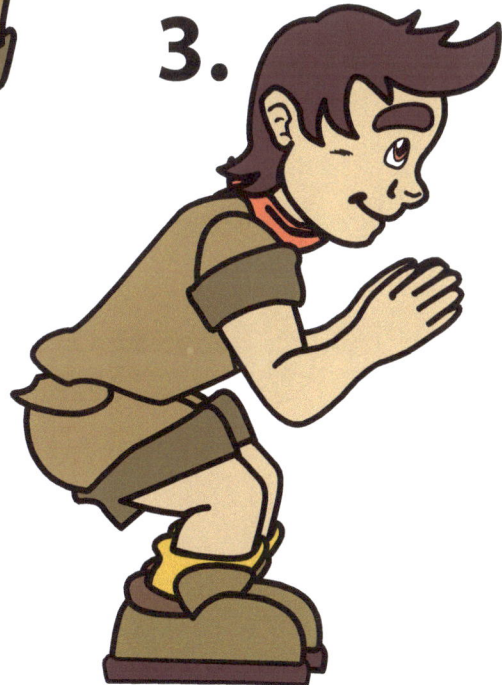

Mountain Climbers

Lie down on the floor

Push your body up

Keep your arms straight and strong

Balance on your arms and feet

Slowly bring one knee up to your chest

Bring it back down again

Can you do this 5 times each side?

1.

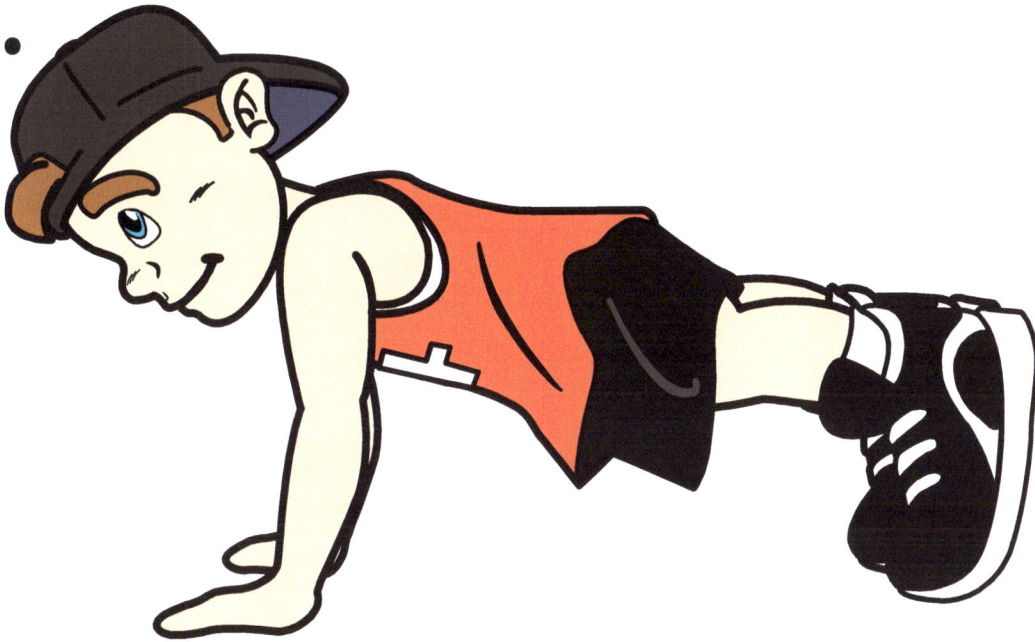

2.

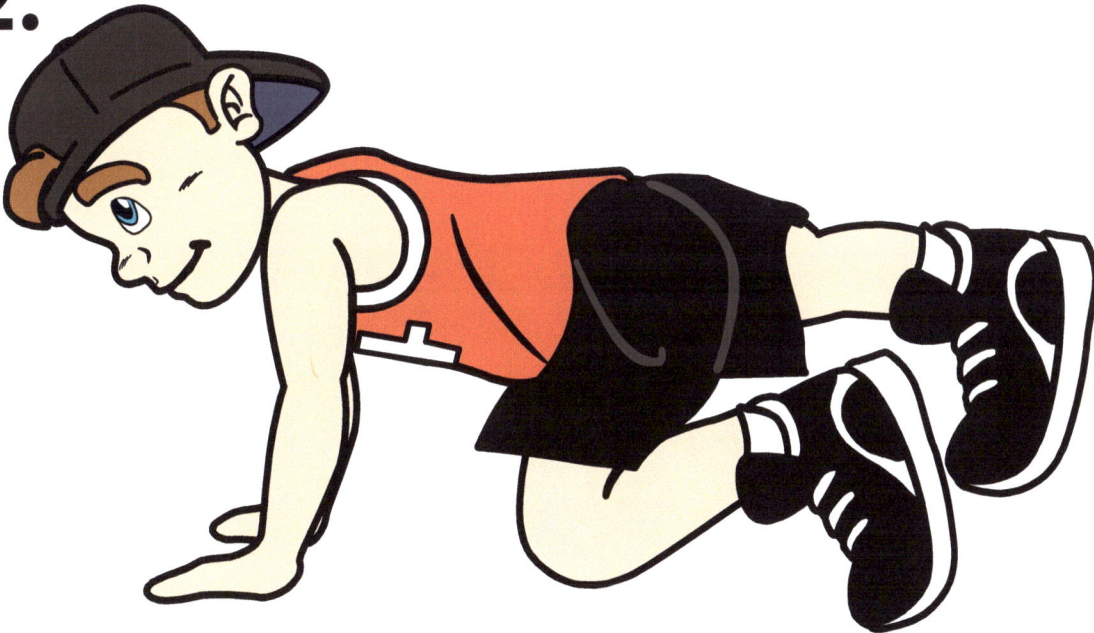

Hook Punches

Put your gloves on your hands

Stand slightly side on with your body

Bring both hands up near your chin

Punch your hand out from the side

Keep your elbows up

Punch one arm from the side at a time

Can you do this 5 times each side?

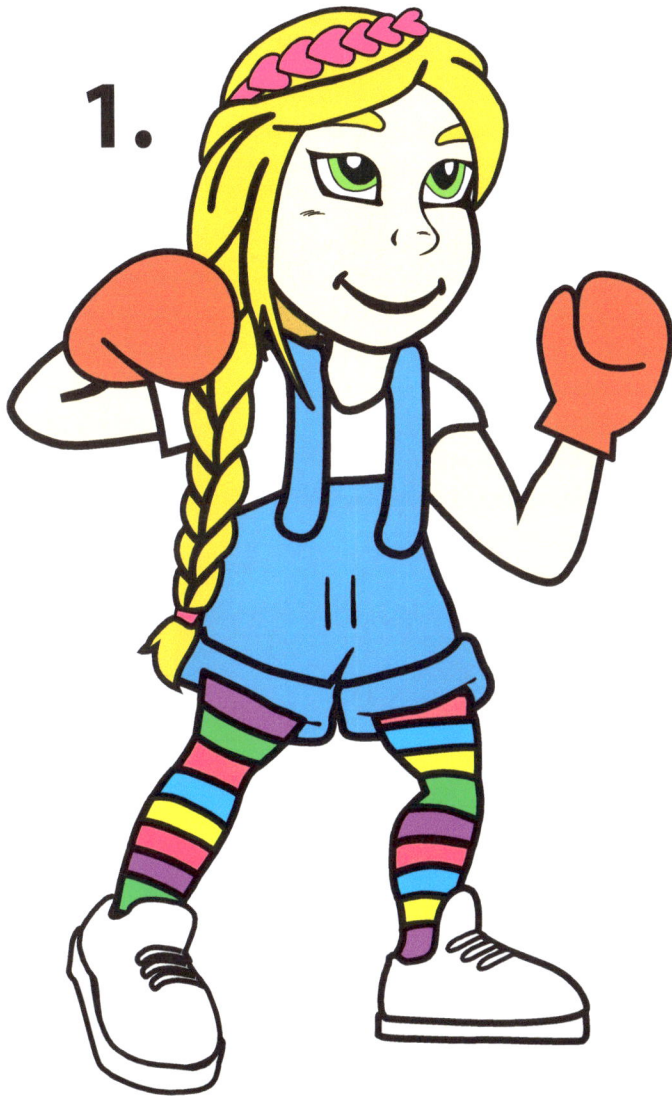

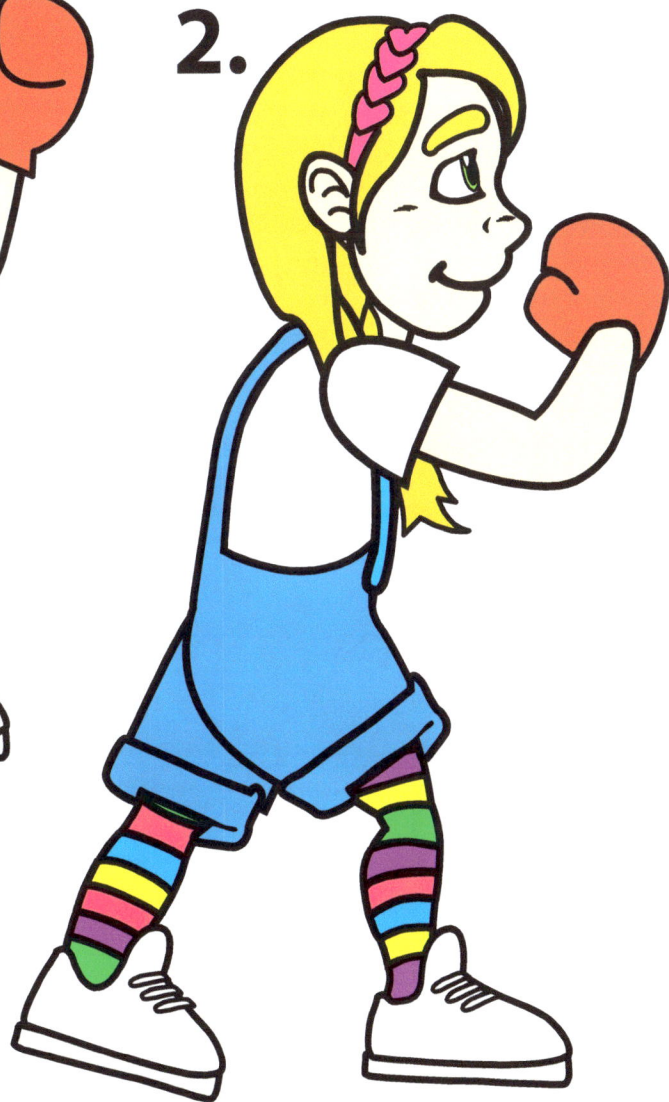

1.

2.

Kick Backs

Stand with your body straight

Bend your elbows

Start swinging them by your sides hip to lip

Start to lift your feet backwards up

towards your bottom

Jog on the spot

Can you do this 5 times each leg?

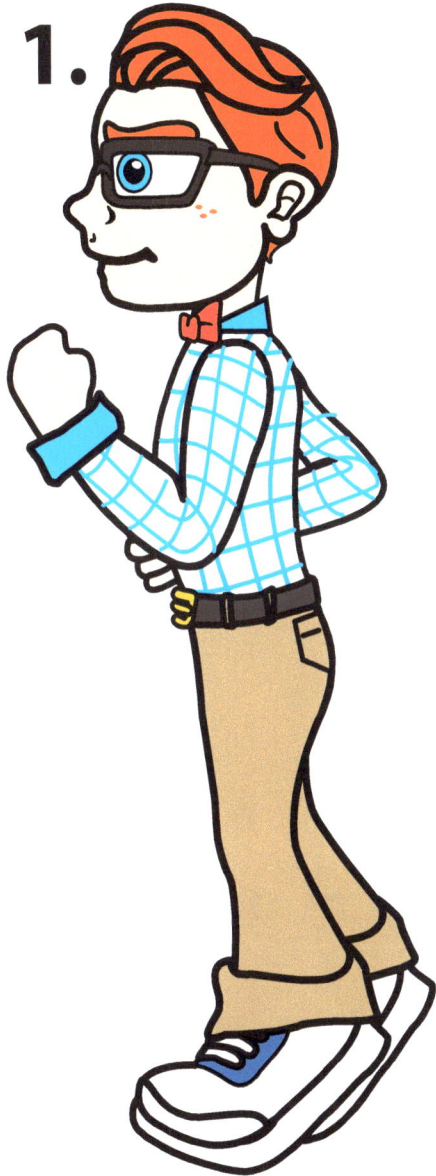

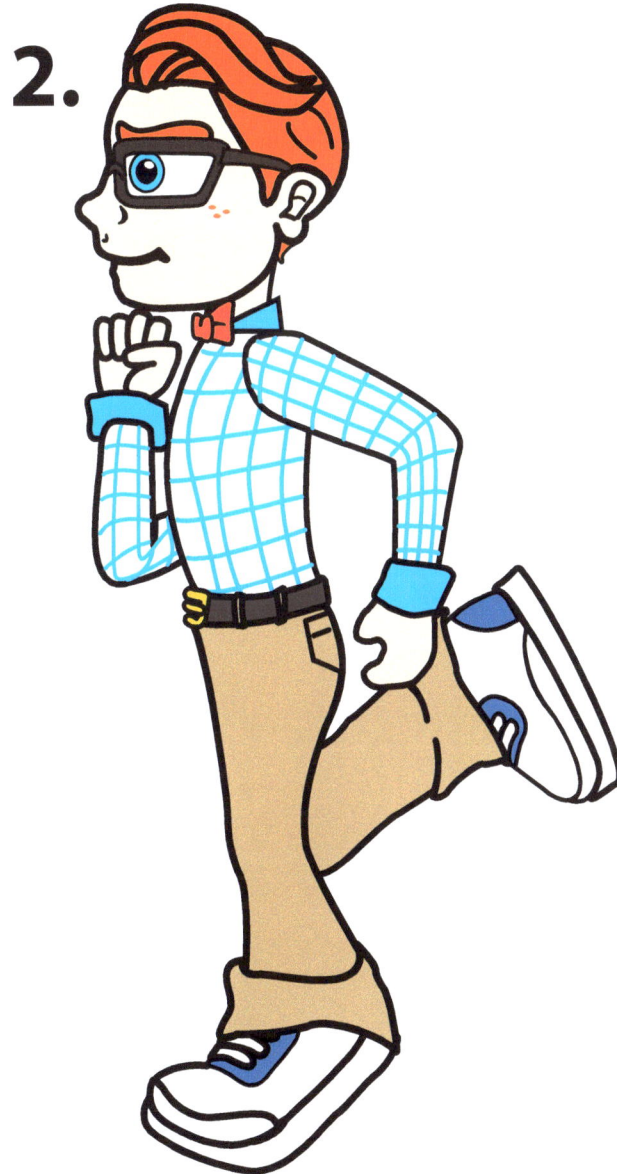

1.

2.

Skipping

Grab your rope

Hold an end at each side

Stand up straight with your feet together

Place the rope behind your feet

Now swing your rope around
your whole body

How many jumps can you do
without stopping?

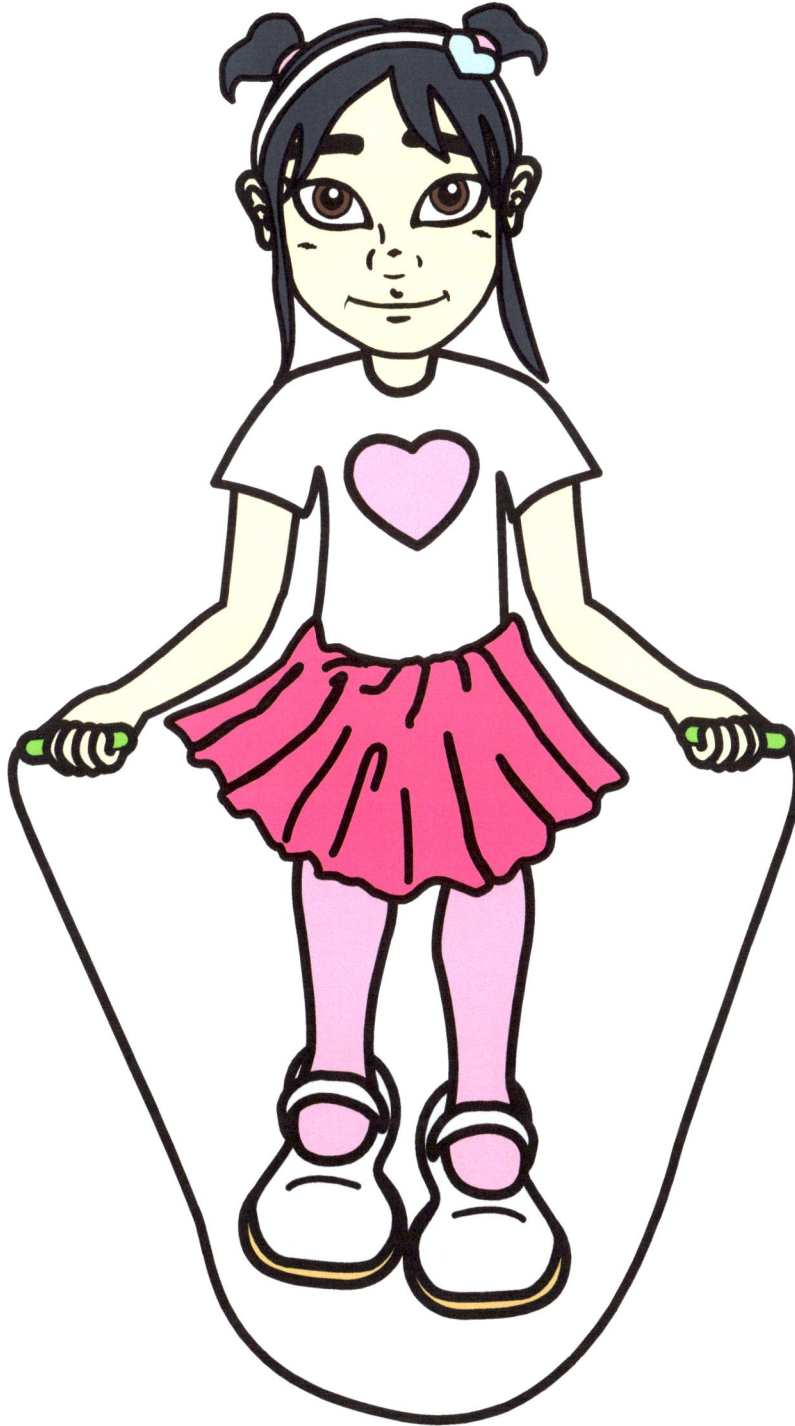

Running

Let's find a big space
Stand with your body straight
Bend your elbows
Start swinging them by your side hip to chin
Start to lift your knees and feet one at a time
Now start to take a step forward
with each leg
Lets see how fast you can run

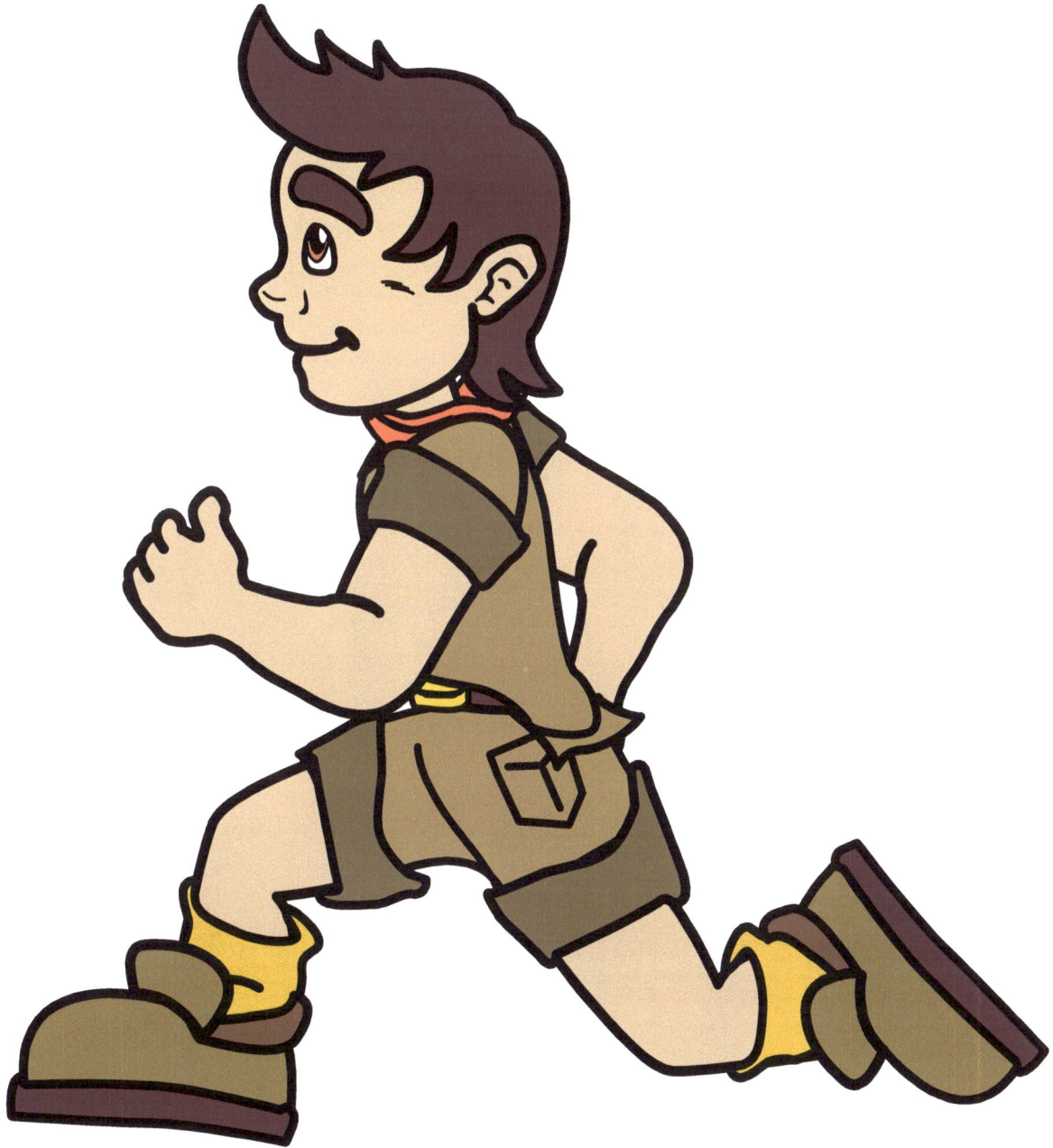

Keep an eye out for the rest of the series

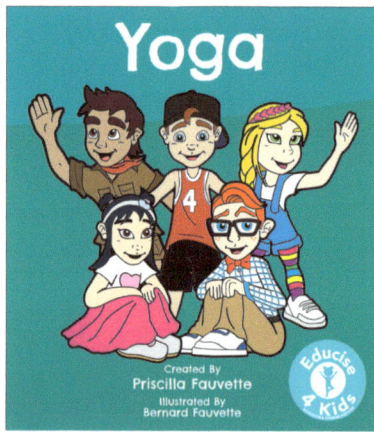

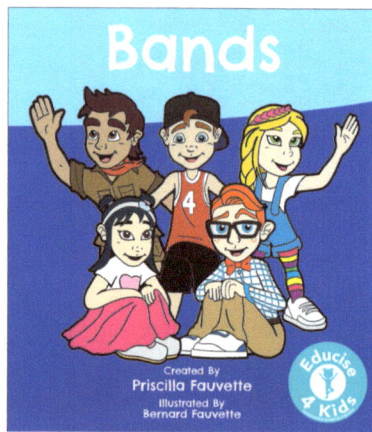

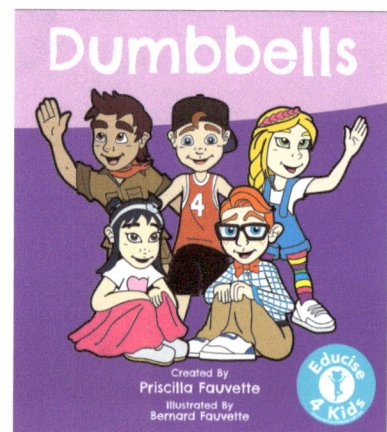

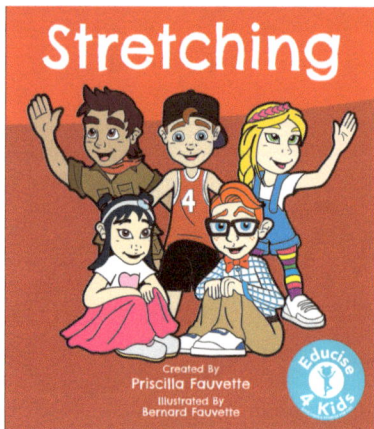

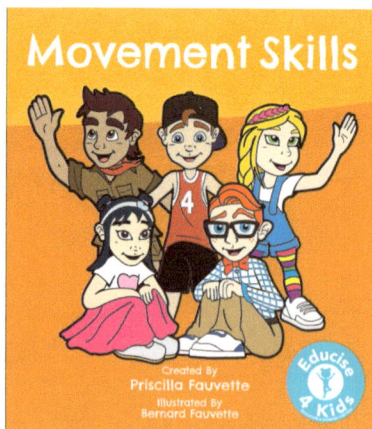

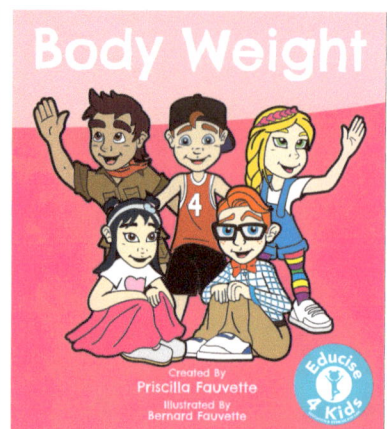

Yoga

Created By
Priscilla Fauvette
Illustrated By
Bernard Fauvette

Educise 4 Kids

Bands

Created By
Priscilla Fauvette
Illustrated By
Bernard Fauvette

Educise 4 Kids

Dumbbells

Created By
Priscilla Fauvette
Illustrated By
Bernard Fauvette

Educise 4 Kids

Stretching

Created By
Priscilla Fauvette
Illustrated By
Bernard Fauvette

Educise 4 Kids

Movement Skills

Created By
Priscilla Fauvette
Illustrated By
Bernard Fauvette

Educise 4 Kids

Body Weight

Created By
Priscilla Fauvette
Illustrated By
Bernard Fauvette

Educise 4 Kids

www.ingramcontent.com/pod-product-compliance
Lightning Source LLC
Chambersburg PA
CBHW061137030426
42334CB00003B/77